# Surviving Braces

# Surviving Braces

*A guide of tips, recipes & more to help you get through orthodontic treatment*

Jennifer Webb and Tracy Gilbert

Created for the office of:

**Note to the reader:**

The information in this book is not meant to be substituted for a doctor's advice. Please use this book as it was intended, as a fun and helpful tool. But don't forget that your orthodontist knows best and you need to consult him or her on all matters concerning your braces.

Surviving Braces
Copyright © 2010 by Surviving Braces LLC

# Table of Contents

**Chapter 3    My Ortho Diary ................4**

# CHAPTER 1

## What to Expect

The first rule of wearing braces is to keep a positive attitude.

Even in the beginning, think about the end and what you are achieving by wearing your braces. Know that your smile is the first impression you make on people – it is your most important asset!

Part of having a positive attitude is being diligent about your treatment. The orthodontist is working for you, providing what you need and guiding you to your perfect smile. You have to do your part too. Wear the appliances and rubber bands, keep your teeth and braces clean, and follow the advice in this book and from your treatment providers.

You are going to love the way you'll look!

## *Can I Get Braces?*

### Can a person be too old to get braces?

**No.** *Anyone that has healthy teeth and gums is able to have their teeth move into new positions. Adults sometimes need a Periodontist to make sure gums are healthy for orthodontic treatment.*

### Can I get braces if I am pregnant?

**Yes.**

### Can I get braces if I have a mouth piercing?

**Yes.**

### Can I get braces if I have crowns?

**Yes.** *Bands and brackets fit the same on crowned teeth as they do regular teeth.*

### Can I get braces if I have a bridge?

**Yes.**

## Can I get braces if I have TMD or TMJ (Jaw Problems)?

> **Yes.** *But you may need to get help with your TMD or TMJ before or during wearing braces. For mild cases, you can wear a splint and be under supervision. For moderate and severe cases you may need to see a specialist, like an Orofacial surgeon to help. Your orthodontist will refer you to a specialist if it is needed.*

## Can I get braces if I am allergic to nickel?

> **Yes.** *Tell your orthodontist if you have an allergy to nickel. There are nickel-free braces and appliances available.*

## The Stages of Getting Braces

In the quest for beautiful teeth, braces are a common cure. Most kids needing orthodontic treatment will start around age eight. About 70% of the teenagers in the US need braces. According to the Consumer Guide to Dentistry, close to 30 percent of all orthodontic patients in the United States are adults.

On your first visit, the orthodontist will examine your mouth to determine if you need orthodontic care.

Questions the orthodontist will be asking himself about your treatment: Is your mouth big enough to hold all of your teeth? Is your palate too narrow? Do you have crooked teeth or teeth that are not in the right place? Do you have missing teeth? When you close your mouth, are the top teeth lined up with your bottom teeth? Are there any other problems like a breathing issue, or a problem with the joint in your jaw? Does your tongue push against your front teeth when you swallow?

The examination is not painful. After the orthodontist looks at you, he will conclude whether you need braces or not.

You may have to wear an appliance before you get braces, which is interceptive treatment. Interceptive treatment is performed to increase the size of your mouth or widen your jaw to make room for your permanent teeth. You may also wear an appliance at the same time you wear braces.

Full orthodontic treatment is the second step. This portion of the treatment continues to extend your mouth and move your teeth around. This is when your braces will be installed.

When your braces are removed, you get a retainer. The retainer is worn 24 hours a day for a period of time, then only night-wear is required. You may get a retainer that is cemented in your mouth. Your orthodontist will decide what is best for you.

## *What does it feel like to get braces?*

**You will feel pressure on your teeth** at first. You may have irritated lips and sores in your mouth. Putting wax between your lip and teeth can help, and rinsing with warm salt water can reduce discomfort.

The first day may not hurt very much. But the **second and third days you may feel discomfort, especially when chewing.** A pain reliever like Ibuprofen (Motrin/Advil) or acetaminophen (Tylenol) can help.

**Soft foods are best to eat at this point.** Consult the recipes (Chapter 6) in this guide to help with this part!

**Chew your food very slowly and carefully.** It will be easy to bite the insides of your cheeks.

**Eating with braces takes some practice.** You may want to run for a mirror to look at your teeth after a meal. After a while, this feeling should subside, but you can carry a small mirror in your purse or pocket to reassure yourself. Brush after meals whenever possible. If brushing is not possible, rinsing with water can help get food out of your braces.

**Use a piece of dental wax on the little hooks or brackets** that hurt. Just break off a piece of wax and put it on the offending spot. If you dry off the braces with a tissue or paper towel, the wax will stay on better.

**Try to get in the habit of flossing once a day.** Your orthodontist assistant will show you the proper flossing technique. There are different kinds of floss to make it easier.

**Your teeth may feel loose after a week or two.** This is normal and will only last a short time.

## *Tips when getting your braces put on*

**Wear lip balm.** Your lips may become dry while your braces are being installed.

**Take a picture.** Get a good photo of yourself before treatment so you can see the changes that are going to take place. Put it in Your *Ortho Diary*, (Chapter 3) in this book!

**If the wire (the archwire) is poking your cheek, tell the assistant so it can be clipped or bent back in place.** This *should not* poke your cheek.

**Can I return to work or school the same day I get braces?** Yes. It should be fine to go to work or school after you get braces, and you typically do not have any side effects. However, at first, you may experience some difficulty speaking with a new appliance. You may also have excess saliva with a new appliance. As soon as your brain adjusts and realizes it is not something to eat, this will subside.

## Clear Aligners

**Clear aligners** use a series of different aligners for top and bottom teeth that are similar in appearance to whitening trays or an athletic mouth guard. Aligners are changed gradually, each new set slightly different from the last, to shift teeth into place.

Aligners must be worn 20 to 22 hours per day, only removing to eat or brush, for treatment to remain on track. Not wearing aligners correctly can set treatment back for *weeks.*

## Tips for Aligners

**Always keep trays in the case while eating.** They can be easily thrown away if wrapped in a napkin.

**Brush your teeth**, or at least rinse with water vigorously, before putting trays back in after eating.

**Only drink water with trays in.** This is the best way to keep aligners clear and undetectable.

**If trays stain** and brushing does not help, you may clean them denture cleaning products. Follow directions on package for best results.

**Bedtime is the best time to change into a new tray**; teeth may be sensitive in a new set of trays. By morning the trays will already feel a little more comfortable. Ibuprofen also helps.

**You may put a water-peroxide solution on cotton swab** to help get stubborn stains, such as lipstick, from aligners. Rub rub it on the stain to remove, then brush aligners with toothpaste.

**Remember that your bite will not always feel "normal."** As with braces your bite is changing daily. This is a normal occurrence.

**Continue reading!** The recommendations in this book are great for any type of orthodontic treatment.

# CHAPTER 2

## Answers and Advice

## *Braces Diagram*

Get to know this information and you can tell your orthodontist, with accuracy, your concerns. Be specific when asking questions about your treatment.

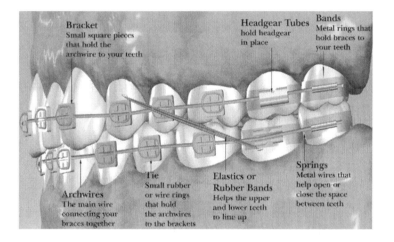

### Terms:

**Bracket** – small square pieces that hold the archwire to your teeth

**Archwire** – the main wire connecting your braces together.

**Tie** – small rubber or wire rings that hold the archwire to the brackets. Can be colored ties.

**Headgear Tubes** – hold headgear in place.

**Bands** – metal rings that hold braces to your teeth.

**Elastics or Rubber Bands** – helps the upper and lower teeth to line up.

**Springs** – metal wires that help open or close the space between teeth.

## *Consider Your Mouth, "Under Construction"*

During treatment it is good to think of your mouth as "under construction." Your teeth will not look straight right away.

Sometimes you may see spaces you have never seen before. A tooth may look out of alignment that used to be straight. All of these things are normal during orthodontic treatment.

Try not to be alarmed and know your smile will look much better soon!

## Some things NOT to eat . . .
### *when you have braces*

Excessive breakage caused by eating the wrong foods can damage braces and appliances and add to treatment time.

Below is a detailed list, but in general what you are trying to avoid are chewy foods, hard foods, crunchy foods and ice.

Ice

Hard candy

Caramel

Taffy

Licorice candy

Hard bread crusts

Pizza crust

Bagels

Hard nuts

Tacos

Tortilla chips

Nuts

Popcorn

Jerky

Corn on the cob

Dried fruit

### Things to make into bite-sized pieces

Raw Carrots – use a vegetable peeler and peel strips of carrots to eat.

Apples – avoid biting into a whole apple.

Steak needs to be cut very small.

Cut corn off of the cob

Tear soft pizza crust in tiny bites

## *Can I Still...?*

### Can I still play a musical instrument like the clarinet, flute or trumpet?

**Yes.** *You can get lip protectors to protect your lips and make it possible for you to still play musical instruments. Wax can also be used to cover your braces when playing an instrument.*

### Can I still play sports if I have braces?

**Yes,** *you can still play football, baseball, basketball, and soccer. You can do anything, but be sure to wear a mouth guard, and try to not get hit in the mouth.*

*Do not use the kind of mouth-guard you boil and fit to your teeth. Your teeth are changing daily. Ask your orthodontist which type of guard is best for you.*

### Can I Snorkel or Scuba Dive with Braces?

*Yes, but be careful with the mouthpieces on the equipment, they can damage your braces.*

## *Tips for Happy Braces*

### Drinking with Braces

**Try to avoid sugary drinks like soft drinks and fruit juices** as much as possible. Stick with water or sugar free drinks because the sugar may cause increased risk of cavities around brackets.

### Pens, Pencils, Fingernails and Braces

**Try not to chew on pens, pencils and fingernails when wearing braces.** This can cause the braces to come loose, leading to added expenses and treatment time.

### Pass up the Urge

**Avoid the urge to play with your braces or appliances with your hands or your tongue.** This will greatly reduce the chance of breakage or bands and brackets coming loose.

It will help to keep your fingers away from your mouth so you will not get in the habit of playing with your braces.

## On Keeping Up Your Dental Care

**Be sure to keep up your regular appointments with your dentist** while you are receiving treatment from the orthodontist.

With braces, your teeth are even more susceptible to bad breath, staining, tooth decay, and gum disease.

Dental hygienists are trained to clean around braces. Keeping your regular dental care going while you wear braces gives you even greater assurance that your teeth will come out looking more beautiful than ever.

If dental work, like fillings or root canals, is required during orthodontic treatment, certain bands or brackets on those teeth can be temporarily removed and replaced after the dental work is complete.

## *Achy Teeth*

The first few days of braces can make teeth feel "achy." The first adjustment will also make your teeth sorer than future adjustments.

**Tips to deal with the achy feelings:**

Spray your teeth and mouth with sore throat spray.

Rinse with warm salt water. Dissolve one teaspoon of salt in an eight ounce glass of warm water and rinse vigorously. Rinse twice a day until you feel better.

Take a pain reliever like ibuprofen (Advil) or acetaminophen (Tylenol).

Rub baby teething gel on gums and teeth.

## *An Irritated Mouth*

Your lips, cheeks and tongue may become irritated as they toughen and become accustomed to the surface of the braces.

Rinse with warm salt water, by following the directions from the previous section.

You can put wax on the braces to make it feel better. But if you can let yourself get through this pain, your cheeks will toughen and not hurt anymore.

It will be helpful for you to learn the difference between roughness that is building calluses in your mouth (something you will have to just let take its course) versus a "wire poking" roughness. Your orthodontic office can help you when a wire is poking or catching your cheek while talking or eating.

## *Waxing Tips*

Orthodontic wax really helps if you have a bracket that is sharp and poking you. It also will come in handy if you have a bracket that is broken.

Just cover the area with wax until you are able to see your orthodontist. **Be sure to dry off the area with a tissue or paper towel first** so the wax will stick better.

If wax is not available, a small piece of wet cotton-ball will work.

## *Keeping Clean*

**Brushing, flossing and rinsing are all *very* important while you are wearing braces.** It is easy for food and plaque to get stuck in braces, wires, springs, rubber bands and other appliances. This will cause bad breath, staining, tooth decay, gum disease or decalcification (permanent white spots on the teeth). Not taking care of your teeth while you are wearing braces can result in *permanent* damage. Your teeth will move easier and faster when your gums are healthy.

**Tips for caring for your teeth while wearing your braces:**

**Brush your teeth after all meals and snacks.**

**To brush your teeth properly,** use a soft toothbrush, and brush in small circles down from the top and up from the bottom of each tooth with braces. Next, use a proxybrush, otherwise known as a "Christmas tree" brush, to clean under the archwire in between the braces. These are sold in drugstores.

**Electric toothbrushes are great for getting braces clean.** But you should be careful not to apply too much pressure with this type of toothbrush to avoid any damage to your braces. Ask your orthodontist for one they recommend.

**Orthodontic technicians are trained to see if the gums are being cleaned properly.** They look for red, swollen gums and plaque build-up. If they see the beginning of a problem, they will again go over brushing techniques with you.

**Floss your teeth daily.**

**To floss with braces,** thread the short end of the floss under the archwire and the upper part of the tooth closest to the gum. Once the floss is under the wire, gently slide it between your teeth. Use an up and down motion on each side of the tooth to remove any food and plaque between the teeth. Gently pull floss from under the archwire and move to the next tooth.

**"Threader" floss, with a stiff end, is good to thread under wire easily.** It is sold in drugstores. Floss threaders can also be used with your regular floss. Ask your technician which is best for you.

**Rinse with a mouthwash.**

**Whether you get one that your orthodontist prescribes or an over-the-counter mouth wash,** it is important to rinse your mouth with a mouthwash to get into places that your brush or floss might not have reached.

**A fluoride rinse works well to help avoid decalcification** of the teeth – white spots – that become permanent stains on the teeth.

## *Wearing Your Rubber Bands*

Rubber bands, or elastics, create tension on your teeth to move them in directions that braces cannot. You need to wear them as prescribed to keep your orthodontic plan on course, because elastics only work if the force is continuous. It is like driving a car uphill. When you take your foot off the gas, it goes back downhill. Skipping days, or even several hours, will slow your treatment.

Change rubber bands several times a day to make sure they keep their elasticity. Remove them only when you brush your teeth or eat, and replace them immediately afterwards.

Wearing your rubber bands as instructed is crucial to receiving the best treatment outcome. If you wear them full time, the soreness they can cause will go away, and it will be easier to wear them.

Your orthodontist can tell if you are not wearing the elastics. A great smile is well worth the effort of wearing them correctly.

## Tips to remember your rubber bands

Try placing small, brightly colored stickers everywhere that you are each day (in your note book, in your locker, in you medicine cabinet etc.). Every time you see that sticker, you will think of rubber bands. This works best if you have a stash of rubber bands in all these places.

Try placing some elastics in several small envelopes and put them *everywhere*. That way, as soon as you remember you don't have to wait to wear them.

Some patients place their elastics around their little finger while eating as a reminder to put them back in after the meal.

Once the elastic soreness subsides, your teeth actually feel better when the elastics are on. When you reach this point, it is easier to remember to wear them. You can do it!

## A Big Elastics No- No

Not wearing your rubber bands for a month then doubling them for a few days before an orthodontic visit will not help and could hurt your treatment outcome. Try to get in the habit right away of wearing the elastics full time.

## A Wire Poking

As your teeth align and spaces and gaps close, the wire that connects your teeth together, the archwire, can actually grow and feel sharp to your cheeks.

This can be frustrating to patients and parents who remember that, "it felt fine when we left."

Try placing wax on the ends of the wire until you can call your orthodontic Office. Usually, a quick wire clip is the only action required.

## A Wire Out
### An At-Home Fix

If the wire comes out of a back brace, sometimes you can place it back into the bracket with tweezers.

If that is not possible, it is alright to try clipping the wire with clean fingernail clippers behind the last bracket that is still securely fastened. Wax can then be placed on the end of the wire for comfort if necessary.

Your orthodontist can repair the wire if you have to cut it. Cutting the wire will not prolong treatment. The rest of your teeth will still move normally.

## *When Things Come Loose*

Don't worry if you realize a bracket is loose on your braces and it is the weekend.

Brackets are held in place by an *elastic tie,* a tiny rubber band (sometimes these are colored ties) that fits around the bracket to hold the archwire in place. This elastic tie should hold the bracket on until you can call your orthodontist.

A bracket on a back tooth can often wait until your regularly scheduled visit with no negative consequences.

### Swallowing Parts of Braces

**Swallowing a piece of your braces is *not* usually a problem.** The parts just pass through your digestive system. This is the same with a separator.

### *Why do I need a retainer?*

Retention Phase is the retainer-wearing part of orthodontic treatment. Teeth are still a little mobile when braces are removed. The retainer holds the teeth still while bone fills in around the new positions of the teeth. It is like how a cast holds a bone immobile while the bone is setting. Without the retainer, your teeth will not stay straight.

This means that if you do not wear the retainer, your teeth can shift back to being uneven. If they shift too much, you could need to wear braces again to have straight teeth. Your orthodontist will prescribe for you the right amount of time you should wear the retainer. Once you get used to wearing a retainer, it is not difficult to wear and it is well worth the effort.

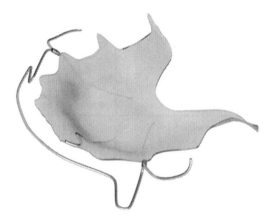

## *Speaking of Appliances*

An orthodontic appliance or retainer may affect your speech at first. A good way to overcome this is to practice reading out loud. This helps train your tongue to use the appliance to speak as you normally would, using the roof of your mouth.

## *Eating with Cemented Appliances*

**When learning to eat with an appliance, cut the food into very small pieces** so you will not have to chew as much.

## *Cleaning a Retainer*

Clean your retainer when you clean your teeth.

Cradle in your hand and brush the acrylic part of the retainer.

Soak it in a denture cleaner at least once a month. Do *not* soak your retainers in mouthwash unless directed by your orthodontist.

Avoid storing them near any source of heat. Do *not* boil your retainer to sterilize it.

For extra cleaning, brush the retainer with an antibacterial soap. Rinse with cool water only!

When possible, rinse off saliva before putting your retainer in its case. This will lessen tartar (calculus) build-up.

## *What if my retainer is too tight?*

A retainer that feels tight usually means more wear is needed. If your orthodontist still has you on full time wear and you are not wearing as instructed, it will be tight. In that case, full time wear is extremely important and necessary.

If your orthodontist has placed you on night wear only and the retainer is getting tight, try putting it in earlier in the evening until it is no longer tight.

### What happens if I swallow a part of the retainer?

Nothing happens. It will pass through your digestive system.

## Challenge: Don't Lose the Appliance

Keeping up with removable appliances is always a challenge. Many trash cans have been sifted through and dumpsters waded through in search of a lost retainer. There's a true story of a mother that went through a school dumpster for an hour before her daughter realized the retainer was in her pocket after all.

If you know you are about to go to lunch, go ahead and remove retainers and put them in the case provided. That way you will not have to take them out at the table, which is where they usually get wrapped in a napkin and thrown in the trash.

Sometimes, thinking ahead is necessary. When going to the movies, amusement parks, or other special places, retainers may be better kept safe in your case than in your mouth.

Get in the habit of carrying your retainer case. Placing a retainer in a pocket without a case will bend and break it.

## *Wrestling with Headgear*

When wearing a headgear appliance, it is a good idea **to *not* roughhouse or wrestle while wearing it.**

Getting hit in the face could damage or bend the appliance. You should remove it when you are running or playing in this manner.

## Communication is Key

Always communicate your concerns with your orthodontic assistant.

If you have had something sharp or loose, or if you have a concern about your elastics, or the way your teeth are progressing tell the assistant. If you notice your gums are red and puffy, the assistant can show you a better brushing technique, or may tell you to brush longer.

Communicating your concerns to the assistant is the key to getting the very best results and a beautiful smile. The orthodontic assistant is there to assist *you*!

## Will it hurt when my braces are removed?

Removal of your braces should not cause any pain. Brackets pop off and are easy to remove.

Next, the orthodontist and assistant will remove adhesive and stains from your teeth.

All of your cooperation and hard work will be worth it when you see your new smile for the first time!

# CHAPTER 3

## My Ortho Diary

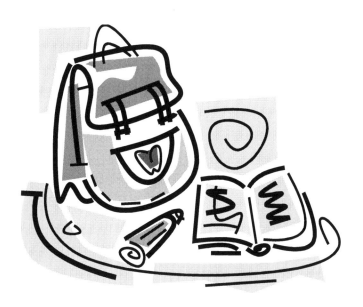

# Photos

Place Your Photo Here

Me Before Braces

Place Your Photo Here

Me After Braces

## My Info

My Orthodontist's Name

_____

_____

_____

Date I started ortho treatment

_____

_____

_____

Date I got my braces put on

_____

_____

_____

Anything special I need to do (like wear rubber bands)?

_____

_____

_____

Date I got my braces off

_____

_____

_____

# How It Feels to Wear an Appliance

## My Appliance(s)

_____

_____

_____

_____

_____

_____

_____

## How it feels

_____

_____

_____

_____

_____

_____

_____

_____

_____

_____

_____

# How It Feels to Have Braces

## First Day

_____

_____

_____

_____

_____

## First Week

_____

_____

_____

_____

_____

## First Month

_____

_____

_____

_____

_____

## First Year

_____

_____

_____

_____

_____

## Elastics Tracker

*You can make a copy of this page and hang it up as a way of tracking your elastics progress. Notice what times you have trouble remembering your elastics and use one of the techniques in the book (        ) to help yourself remember them.*

**Day 1** _____ Rubber Bands In

Changed _____

Changed _____

Changed _____

Changed _____

Changed _____

Changed _____

**Day 2** _____ Rubber Bands In

Changed _____

Changed _____

Changed _____

Changed _____

Changed _____

Changed _____

**Day 3** _____ Rubber Bands In

Changed _____

Changed _____

Changed _____

Changed _____

Changed _____

Changed _____

**Day 4** _____ Rubber Bands In

Changed _____

Changed _____

Changed _____

Changed _____

Changed _____

Changed _____

**Day 5** _____ Rubber Bands In

Changed _____

Changed _____

Changed _____

Changed _____

Changed _____

Changed _____

**Day 6** _____ Rubber Bands In

Changed _____

Changed _____

Changed _____

Changed _____

Changed _____

Changed _____

**Day 7** _____ Rubber Bands In

Changed _____

Changed _____

Changed _____

Changed _____

Changed _____

Changed _____

## Sharing Braces

Friends wearing braces at the same time as me

_____

_____

_____

_____

_____

_____

_____

_____

_____

Celebrities wearing braces at the same time as me

_____

_____

_____

_____

_____

_____

_____

_____

_____

# Eating With Braces

My favorite "braces" food(s)

_____

_____

_____

_____

_____

_____

_____

_____

_____

_____

_____

_____

_____

_____

_____

_____

_____

_____

_____

_____

_____

_____

_____

## My Braces Are Off!

What it means to me that I accomplished orthodontic treatment

_____

_____

_____

_____

_____

_____

_____

_____

_____

_____

_____

_____

_____

_____

_____

_____

_____

_____

_____

_____

_____

_____

# My Retainer

## First Day

_____

_____

_____

_____

## First Week

_____

_____

_____

_____

## First Month

_____

_____

_____

_____

## First Year

_____

_____

_____

_____

# CHAPTER 4

## Been There, Done That

In this chapter you will find experiences and advice from others that have worn appliances.

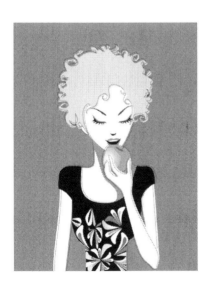

## Tongue Habit Appliance

Karla Martinez, age 19

♦ What was the most challenging part of wearing the Tongue Habit appliance?

Answer: *Being able to speak and swallow normally. At first eating was hard.*

♦ How did you get through these challenges?

Answer: *I practiced swallowing with my tongue behind the appliance.*

♦ How long did it take for you to get used to the appliance?

Answer: *It took about two weeks to speak clearly and to be comfortable.*

♦ What foods were the easiest to eat while wearing the appliance?

Answer: *Mashed potatoes, cooked soft vegetables, soups*

♦ Do you have any advice for patients that have this type of appliance?

Answer: *My teeth look really good now after my treatment. Hang in there, it is worth it. I now have a tongue habit appliance made into my retainer to help me keep my tongue back.*

## Arch Expander

Riley Ware, age 9

♦ What was the most challenging part of wearing the Arch Expander?

Answer: *Eating with it was the hardest part.*

♦ How did you get through these challenges?

Answer: *I used small proxy brush to help clean it after meals.*

♦ How long did it take for you to get used to the appliance?

Answer: *By two weeks I wasn't complaining as much, my mom says!*

♦ What foods were the easiest to eat while wearing the appliance?

Answer: *Mashed potatoes, pasta, ice cream*

♦ Do you have any advice for patients that have this type of appliance?

Answer: *Try to remember you do not have to have your appliance in for very long. It is great to get it out!*

### Elastics

Amy Gangi, age 28

♦ What was the most challenging part of wearing Elastics?

Answer: *The pain and getting the elastics on my braces correctly.*

♦ How did you get through these challenges?

Answer: *I was in pain for about a week but I continued to wear them consistently and took Advil. After about a week or two I could put them on easier because I changed them four to five times a day.*

♦ How long did it take for you to get used to the appliance?

Answer: *About a week.*

♦ What foods were the easiest to eat while wearing the appliance?

Answer: *Does not apply. I took them out when I ate.*

♦ Do you have any advice for patients that have this type of appliance?

Answer: *Be consistent and the pain won't last.*

## Herbst

Courteney Welch, age 15

♦ What was the most challenging part of wearing the Herbst appliance?

Answer: *Eating, talking and brushing my teeth. Getting used to the bulk of the appliance beside my lip.*

♦ How did you get through these challenges?

Answer: *Soft foods cut up very small. Wax, wax and more wax! Rinsed with salt water.*

♦ How long did it take for you to get used to the appliance?

Answer: *A couple of weeks to get used to eating and talking. Wax placed on the appliance helped my lips get used to it.*

♦ What foods were the easiest to eat while wearing the appliance?

Answer: *Mashed potatoes, mac and cheese, shredded chicken casseroles, scrambled eggs, and soups.*

♦ Do you have any advice for patients that have this type of appliance?

Answer: *Try not to get discouraged. Keep clean so your lips will not get as irritated.*

### Expander and Braces

Madison Woodward, age 14

♦ What was the most challenging part of wearing the Expander appliance and Braces?

Answer: *The worst thing about the expander was learning to speak with it. I sounded like a creepy elf.*

♦ How did you get through these challenges?

Answer: *I practiced saying as many tongue-twisters as I could until I learned to say every word correctly.*

♦ How long did it take for you to get used to the appliance?

Answer: *About three weeks. It took less time for me to stop laughing at how I sounded. My mom even got a kick out of it!*

♦ What foods were the easiest to eat while wearing the appliance?

Answer: *Milk shakes. Never try eating sushi with one unless you want to be cleaning it out for the next three days!*

♦ Do you have any advice for patients that have this type of appliance?

Answer: *Stay away from sticky foods. Cut carrots and apples into small pieces to eat. Brush at least two or three times a day.*

## Retainer

Tyler Ward, age 17

♦ What was the most challenging part of wearing the Retainer?

Answer: *Talking in it was hard. It made me have a lot of saliva in my mouth.*

♦ How did you get through these challenges?

Answer: *I practiced reading out loud to train my tongue to speak clearly.*

♦ How long did it take for you to get used to the appliance?

Answer: *Within a few days I could speak clearly. The saliva lessened when my brain realized the retainer wasn't food!*

♦ What foods were the easiest to eat while wearing the appliance?

Answer: *Does not apply. You take the retainer out to eat.*

♦ Do you have any advice for patients that have this type of appliance?

Answer: *Don't take it out when you talk – just practice.*

## Distalizer

Sara Taylor, age 14

♦ What was the most challenging part of wearing the Distalizer appliance?

Answer: *Eating! Food always got stuck in it.*

♦ How did you get through these challenges?

Answer: *I drank a lot of milk shakes. I threaded floss under the appliance to get food out.*

♦ How long did it take for you to get used to the appliance?

Answer: *About one month. I practiced reading out loud to train my tongue and it really helped me to talk clearly.*

♦ What foods were the easiest to eat while wearing the appliance?

Answer: *Ice cream and yogurt.*

♦ Do you have any advice for patients that have this type of appliance?

Answer: *Just be patient and eat a lot of ice cream!*

## Headgear Appliance

Nathan Johnson, age 13

♦ What was the most challenging part of wearing the Headgear appliance?

Answer: *Getting used to sleeping in it.*

♦ How did you get through these challenges?

Answer: *I found the best position to sleep on was my back. I also found I could sleep on my side if I cupped my hand around the appliance.*

♦ How long did it take for you to get used to the appliance?

Answer: *About three weeks.*

♦ What foods were the easiest to eat while wearing the appliance?

Answer: *Does not apply. You take it off to eat.*

♦ Do you have any advice for patients that have this type of appliance?

Answer: *My advice would be to wear it as much as possible while at home during the day if it is too difficult to sleep in at night.*

# CHAPTER 5

## On a Lighter Note

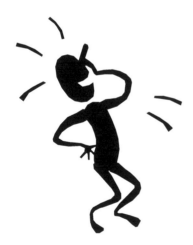

## Where did braces come from?
### A brief history of orthodontics

According to the American Association of Orthodontists, ancient Romans and mummified ancients were discovered with metal and wires on their teeth thought to be used as an attempt at straightening them.

But orthodontics really advanced in the 1700s when a French dentist named Pierre Fauchard published his book, "The Surgeon Dentist." After that, many different people built upon the next to make modern orthodontic treatment available.

The first set of braces, made in the 1900s, was made of gold. Talk about expensive!

Now orthodontists use heat activated wires developed by NASA. Another technology available uses clear trays to be worn progressively to move the teeth into position without braces.

## How to Become an Orthodontist

An orthodontist needs four years of college, four years of dental school and two to three years of postgraduate study in orthodontics before they can practice orthodontics.

All orthodontists are board certified dentists.

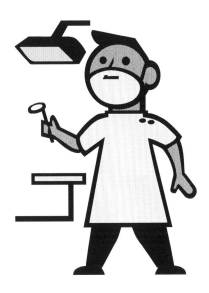

## Humor from the Chair
## Stories told by Orthodontic Assistants

Once when calling an apprehensive patient to the back the doctor said, "Please put him in the *consultation* room."

The patient looked horrified and said, "No! I don't want to go to the *complication* room!"
— **Melody Jordan**

I once had a little girl in the chair. I was setting up for her x-rays and impressions that we call pre-treatment records.

As I started explaining the procedures she looked at me with such disappointment. I asked her what was wrong. "Oh nothing, my mom said if I came back here all I would have to do is listen to some records."
— **Kelly Woodward**

In orthodontics, I guess some of our appliances can look pretty strange, especially through the eyes of a child. Once, a patient's three-year-old sister came with mom to hear instructions given for an expansion appliance.

Seeing everyone peer down at something in my hand made her curious. "Let me see," she said. I bent to let her look at the odd shaped appliance.

"Oooo" she said softly, "Put it down and see if it will walk."

**— Amy Gangi**

Once I was seating a patient who seemed a little apprehensive. Being that she was an older lady, I tried to reassure her that our practice was not only for children but adults as well.

She sat down and looked at the wall and said, "But Miss, why do you have all these pictures of teeth on the wall?"

I assured her that many orthodontists show pictures of their work.

She looked at me in embarrassment as she jumped up from the chair and said, "Orthodontists! I thought this was an Ophthalmologist!"

Being that there was an Ophthalmologist with the same last name nearby, I'm surprised it didn't happen more often.

**— Tracy Gilbert**

A teen patient was in the chair and had just gotten her braces. Her four-year-old brother moved closer to the chair and looked at her braces curiously.

As they were about to leave, he was touching his own teeth like he was trying to make one loose. "What are you doing?" asked his mother. He looked up at her seriously and said, "I am fixing *my* teeth so I can get bracelets!'"

— **Betty Phillips**

Once a little girl came in who was distressed because she had a loose bracket. It was her third loose bracket that month. "What were you doing to make your bracket come off?" I asked.

"I wasn't doing anything but sitting on the couch," said the patient.

I jokingly replied, "Well if that couch makes your braces loose maybe you should sit somewhere else."

The next time the patient came in I was glad to see no braces were broken. "What did you do different?" I asked.

The little girl looked at me seriously and said, "I sat on the chair instead of the couch."

— **Betty Phillips**

Once, at the end of a long day, it was time to call in the last patient. As I walked down the hall, I glanced down at the chart and saw her last name was Presley.

I entered the reception area, and for some reason, that to this day I can't understand, called out loudly and clearly, "ELVIS!"

As soon as it came out of my mouth I wanted to die of embarrassment! The room full of people looked at me with puzzled expressions. I slowly turned around and walked back down the hall, grabbed a coworker and asked her to please go and call the patient by her correct name. We still laugh about it to this day.

— **Tracy Gilbert**

### *Funny Things Can Happen to Retainers*

Some reasons given when asked, *"How did you lose your retainer?"*

"The ocean hit me in the face and took it."

"My dog thought it was something to eat."

"It was under my bed and the vacuum got it."

"I was turning cartwheels and it must have fallen out of my pocket."

"I left it in the yard and my dad found it with the lawnmower."

"My toddler flushed it down the toilet."

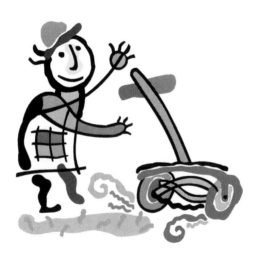

## *Just a Few Famous People that Have Worn Braces*

Michael Jordan

Cher (wore braces as an adult)

Chelsea Clinton

Cindy Crawford

Cameron Diaz

Brett Favre

Jodie Foster

Woopie Goldberg

Prince Harry of England

Caroline Kennedy

Nancy Kerrigan

Anna Kournikova

Heather Locklear

Allysa Milano

Diana Ross (worn as an adult)

Monica Seles

Barbara Walters (worn as an adult)

Serena and Venus Williams

Kristi Yamaguccia

# CHAPTER 6

## Recipes

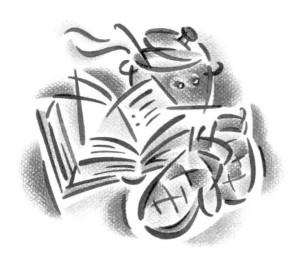

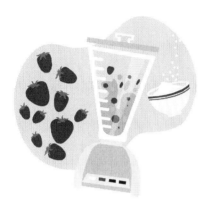

# Smoothies and Milk Shakes

Smoothies and milk shakes are great options for you to drink at the beginning of wearing braces. When your teeth hurt and you are hungry, you need the softest of foods.

Smoothies, if you make them with healthful ingredients, can have plenty of nutrition packed in these delicious concoctions to keep you healthy, while your mouth gets used to your new braces.

## Smoothie Tips

**A good order of ingredients goes like this**: liquid, frozen fruit, powders, ice, and then fresh fruit. The ice is on top because if it is on bottom it can be over-blended and make the smoothie watery.

**Common liquid bases** for smoothies are fruit juices such as pineapple, apple and orange. But don't be afraid to get creative. Some other choices could be: green tea, coffee, coconut juice, carrot juice, pomegranate juice, milk (cow's, soy, almond or goat's milk, are all good), yogurt and plain old water.

**Make ice cubes from your liquid** to use as your ice to avoid using too much ice in your smoothie. It makes for a richer flavor and a thicker smoothie.

**Frozen fruit is the best way to use fruit** in a smoothie, even if you buy fresh fruit and freeze it yourself. When freezing bananas, be sure to peel and chop the banana first. Fresh, unfrozen fruit is still a great addition to a smoothie. But, put it in last (so it doesn't get too pulverized before the frozen stuff).

It is best to put less liquid in a smoothie in the beginning. You can always add more liquid later, but you can't take it out.

A few healthy additions to your smoothie can be flax seed, wheat germ or ground nuts, like almonds, walnuts, cashews or peanuts. These ingredients increase fiber. In the case of flaxseed and walnuts these ingredients add omega-3 oils we all need.

Protein powders are available in health food and grocery stores to increase the protein of your smoothies and keep your appetite satisfied longer.

Other ingredients that might not come to mind at first but make great additions are peanut butter, tofu (adds creaminess to a smoothie) or cooked oatmeal.

To save time on making smoothies you can make a large batch and freeze some for later. Let it thaw in the fridge for about an hour before you are ready to drink.

A blender, smoothie maker or a food processor are the only equipment necessary for a smoothie – you pick the one that works best for you!

## Orange Banana Cream Smoothie

¼ cup milk (any kind of milk)
½ cup orange juice
dash of vanilla
½ frozen banana (chunks)
½ cup vanilla frozen yogurt

Pour all liquid ingredients into the blender. Add all frozen ingredients. Blend 30 seconds or until desired consistency.

## Blueberry-Banana Smoothie

½ cup milk
¾ cup yogurt
1 cup frozen blueberries
½ frozen or fresh banana
1 scoop protein powder (optional)
1 cup ice

Put liquid ingredients into blender. Add protein powder. Add all frozen ingredients and blend until desired consistency.

## A Banana-Berry Good Smoothie

> ½ cup nonfat milk
> ½ cup fat-free plain yogurt
> ½ frozen banana, peeled and chopped
> 2 tablespoons powdered protein supplement (optional)
> 1 ½ tablespoons flax seed or flax seed oil
> ½ cup frozen strawberries

Put liquid ingredients into blender. Add protein powder and flax seed or oil. Add all frozen ingredients and blend until desired consistency.


## Mango-Cherry Smoothie

> ½ cup pineapple juice
> ½ cup frozen cherries
> ½ cup frozen mango
> 1 scoop powdered protein supplement (optional)
> ½ cup ice

Put liquid ingredients into blender. Add protein powder. Add all frozen ingredients and blend until desired consistency.

## Drink Your Greens Smoothie

1 frozen banana, cut in chunks
1 cup grapes
1 (6 ounce) cup vanilla yogurt
½ apple, peeled, cored and chopped
1 ½ cups fresh spinach leaves
½ cup of ice

Put yogurt into blender. Add all frozen ingredients. Add apples, grapes and spinach (in that order). Blend until desired consistency.

## Mango-Peach Smoothie

½ cup vanilla soy milk
½ cup orange juice, or as needed
1 peach, sliced or 1 cup frozen peach slices
1 mango, peeled and diced or 1 cup frozen mango chunks
½ cup of ice

Put liquid ingredients into blender. Add all frozen ingredients. Add Fresh fruit. Blend until desired consistency.

## Orange-Vanilla Banana Smoothie

1 cup orange juice
1 frozen banana
½ cup vanilla fat-free yogurt *or* 1 scoop vanilla protein powder
½ cup cubes ice

Put liquid ingredients into blender. Add protein powder (if using). Add all frozen ingredients and blend until desired consistency.

## Chocolate-Banana Smoothie

1 frozen banana
2-3 tablespoons chocolate syrup
1 cup milk
½ cup crushed ice

Put liquid ingredients into blender. Add chocolate syrup. Add frozen ingredients and blend until desired consistency.

## Cranberry-Banana Smoothie

¼ cup cranberry Juice
¾ cup milk
¼ cup frozen blueberries
½ frozen banana
1 tablespoon honey
2-3 ice cubes

Put liquid ingredients into blender. Add honey. Add all frozen ingredients. Blend until desired consistency.

## Coconut-Orange Smoothie

1 cup orange juice
2 cups coconut milk (better if you pre-make ice cubes with the milk, or coconut juice)
1 frozen banana

Put liquid ingredients into blender. Add frozen banana. Blend until desired consistency.

## Blueberry Blast Smoothie

1 cup pineapple juice or water
1 serving vanilla protein powder
1 cup frozen blueberries
4 ice cubes

Put liquid ingredients into blender. Add protein powder. Add all frozen ingredients and blend until desired consistency.

## Chocolate Coffee Smoothie

1 cup milk
½ cup of water
1 serving chocolate protein powder
1 tablespoon instant coffee
4-6 ice cubes

Put liquid ingredients into blender. Add protein powder and instant coffee. Add all frozen ingredients. Blend until desired consistency.

## Whipped Raspberry Surprise

1 cup apple juice
¼ cup cottage cheese
1 teaspoon honey
1 cup frozen raspberries

Put liquid ingredients into blender. Add cottage cheese and honey. Add frozen raspberries. Blend until desired consistency.

## Banana Oatmeal Smoothie

1 cup apple juice
½ cup milk
3 tablespoons uncooked oatmeal
2 tablespoons honey
1 frozen banana
4 ice cubes

Put liquid ingredients into blender. Add oatmeal and honey. Add frozen ingredients. Blend until desired consistency.

## Groovy Smoothie

½ cup orange juice
1 (8 ounce) container vanilla yogurt
1 kiwi, sliced
1 frozen banana
½ cup frozen or fresh blueberries
1 cup frozen or fresh strawberries
1 cup frozen or fresh peaches (can substitute peach yogurt)
1 cup ice cubes

Put liquid ingredients into blender. Add all frozen ingredients. Add fresh fruit. Blend until desired consistency.

## Happy Mango Smoothie

1 cup orange juice
1 cup vanilla nonfat yogurt
1 cup frozen mango (or fresh copped into chunks)
1 frozen banana
½ cup ice

Put liquid ingredients into blender. Add all frozen ingredients and blend until desired consistency.

## Milk Shake Tips

**A good order of ingredients goes like this**: milk, ice cream and other ingredients like yogurt, creams and fruit.

**Less milk is better to start** with for a creamier milk shake. You can always add more milk at the end to make it less thick.

**Use premium ice cream** for better taste.

**Use fresh fruit for a better flavor.** Frozen fruit will enhance the creamy texture of your shake.

**Be creative with your ingredients.** If you have pie, cheesecake, cookies, or other dessert items, throw them in a shake with some chocolate ice cream or anything that sounds good to you.

## Basic Vanilla Milk Shake

*Start with this basic shake then add creative ingredients; bananas, orange juice, strawberries, blueberries or chocolate syrup – the options are endless!*

> 2 cups vanilla ice cream
> ½ cup whole milk
> 1 teaspoon vanilla extract

### Directions

In a blender, combine ice cream, milk and vanilla extract. Blend until smooth. Pour into glasses and serve.

## Basic Chocolate Shake

*Start with this chocolate milkshake. Then, once again, get creative; add a shot of espresso, bananas, raspberries, peanut butter or brownies – you decide what will make you happy.*

2 cups chocolate ice cream
¼ cup whole milk
¼ cup of chocolate syrup or chocolate powdered drink mix

### Directions

In a blender, combine ice cream, milk and syrup or powder mix. Blend until smooth. Add ¼ cup more milk if it is too thick for your taste, stir. Pour into glasses and serve.

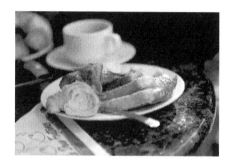

# Breakfast Foods

## Cheesy Basil Scrambled Eggs

4 eggs
3 tablespoons sour cream
½ cup shredded mozzarella cheese
salt and pepper to taste
2 teaspoons butter
1 tablespoon minced fresh basil (or any herb of your choice)

### Directions

Whisk eggs and sour cream in a bowl until creamy and smooth. Mix in cheese. Season with salt and pepper.

Melt butter in a skillet over medium heat. Pour in egg mixture; cook, stirring constantly, until eggs reach the desired consistency. Mix in basil during final minutes of cooking.

## Spinach-Feta Frittata

5 eggs
¾ cup of cottage cheese
¼ cup of feta cheese
1 package of sliced portabella mushrooms
¼ or ½ cup onion
1 cup fresh spinach
1 teaspoon butter

**Directions**

Preheat oven to 375°.

In a skillet on medium-high heat sauté onion in a teaspoon of butter. Add mushrooms and cook until tender. At the end, put in spinach and wilt it, about 2-3 minutes.

In a bowl, mix or whisk the eggs, cottage cheese and feta cheese together in a bowl, add in the spinach mixture and mix everything together.

Pour in a greased pie pan and bake for 30 minutes or until the top starts to brown.

## Quick Quiche

*Add any meat or veggies to this recipe to make it your way. This is the "plain" version to make it braces friendly in the beginning.*

> ½ cup shredded Swiss cheese
> ½ cup cheddar cheese
> 4 eggs, beaten
> ¼ cup finely chopped onion
> 1 teaspoon salt
> ½ cup all-purpose flour
> 1 ½ cups milk

### Directions

Preheat oven to 350 ° (175 degrees C).

Lightly grease a 9 inch pie pan.

Line the bottom of the pie plate with Swiss and cheddar cheeses.

In a bowl, combine eggs, onion, salt, flour and milk; whisk together until smooth; pour into pie pan.

Bake in preheated oven for 35 minutes, until set. Serve hot or cold.

# French Toast Casserole

5 cups bread cubes (use soft bread or soak a hard bread in mixture overnight)
4 eggs
1 ½ cups milk
¼ cup white sugar, divided
¼ teaspoon salt
1 teaspoon vanilla extract
1 tablespoon margarine, softened
2 teaspoon ground cinnamon
½ teaspoon ground nutmeg

## Directions

Preheat oven to 350 °.

Lightly butter an 8x8 inch baking pan.

Line bottom of pan with bread. In a large bowl, beat together eggs, milk, 2 tablespoons sugar, salt and vanilla. Pour egg mixture over bread. Dot with margarine; let stand for 10 minutes.

Combine remaining 2 tablespoons sugar with cinnamon and nutmeg and sprinkle over the top. Bake in preheated oven about 60 minutes, until top is golden.

## Just Peachy Pancakes

4 eggs
1 cup cottage cheese
½ cup milk
1 teaspoon vanilla extract
2 tablespoons butter, melted
1 peach, shredded
1 cup all-purpose flour
2 tablespoons white sugar
1 pinch salt
¾ teaspoon baking soda
1 heaping teaspoon ground cinnamon

### Directions

Mix eggs, cottage cheese, milk, vanilla, butter, and peach in a large bowl. Combine flour, sugar, salt, baking soda, and cinnamon in a small bowl. Stir flour mixture into the cottage cheese mixture until just combined.

Heat a lightly oiled griddle over medium-high heat. Drop batter by large spoonfuls onto the griddle, and cook until bubbles form and the edges are dry. Flip, and cook until browned on the other side. Repeat with remaining batter.

# Baby Bear's Porridge

*This is a filling meal. Eat this when your teeth hurt to give you more time between meals and less pain to your mouth.*

3 cups water
1 cup powdered milk
1 ½ cups rolled oats
¾ teaspoon ground cinnamon
½ teaspoon vanilla extract
3 eggs
4 teaspoons butter
1 cup milk
3 tablespoons honey

## Directions

In a large saucepan, bring the water to a boil.

Combine the powdered milk, oats and cinnamon. Quickly stir into the boiling water.

Return the mixture to a boil, then reduce heat and simmer for 5 to 10 minutes, or until the mixture is the desired thickness.

Keep heat low and mix in vanilla. Beat in the eggs one at a time, mixing well after each. Make sure eggs are cooked.

Divide the porridge between 4 bowls. Top each one with a teaspoon of butter, 1/4 cup of milk, and drizzle with honey.

## Grandma's Oatmeal

*Mushy cold cereal, hot cereal and oatmeal are good meals for sore teeth.*

3 ¾ cups water
2 cups rolled oats
1 pinch salt
4 teaspoons butter
¼ cup brown sugar
1 cup non-dairy creamer
4 tablespoons milk
¼ cup brown sugar

### Directions

In a medium saucepan, heat water to boiling.

Reduce heat to low; stir in oats and salt. Cook until oats have thickened, about 5 minutes.

Place 1 teaspoon of butter and 1 tablespoon of brown sugar in the bottom of each four serving bowls.

Spoon oatmeal into each bowl and stir until butter and sugar are melted. Pour 1/4 cup of creamer and 1 tablespoon of milk over each bowl.

Top each serving with another tablespoon of brown sugar. Serve hot.

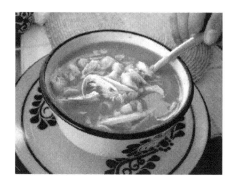

# Soups

## Broccoli Cheese Soup

1 medium onion, chopped
1 tablespoon margarine
6 cups chicken broth
1 (8 ounce) package wide egg noodles
24 ounce bag frozen chopped broccoli
1 clove garlic, minced
4 cups milk or half and half (for thicker soup)
1 ½ cup shredded American cheese
1 cup shredded cheddar cheese

### Directions

In a large saucepan, sauté onion and garlic in butter or margarine over medium heat until tender. Add broth, and bring to a boil. Reduce heat, and add noodles. Cook for 3 to 4 minutes. Stir in broccoli. Cover, and cook for 5 minutes.

Stir in milk and cheese. Heat slowly, stirring, till cheese melts. DO NOT BOIL. Serve immediately.

## Curry Carrot Soup

2 tablespoons vegetable oil
1 onion, chopped
1 clove garlic, minced
1 ½ tablespoon curry powder
2 pounds carrots, chopped
5 cups vegetable broth
2 cups water, or as needed
Salt to taste, recommend starting with ¼ teaspoon

### Directions

Heat oil in a large pot over medium heat. Sauté onion and garlic until tender. Stir in the curry powder. Add the chopped carrots, and stir until the carrots are coated.

Pour in the vegetable broth, and simmer until the carrots are soft, about 25 minutes.

Transfer the carrots and broth to a blender, and puree until smooth. Pour back into the pot, and thin with water to your preferred consistency. Salt to your taste.

## Chicken Corn Chowder

3 breasts
1 chicken flavored bouillon cube
1 onion, chopped
3 potatoes, diced small
½ bag of frozen yellow corn
8 oz. package of Velveeta Cheese

### Directions

In a medium pot, place bouillon cube and onion and boil chicken breast until tender and cooked through, about 20 minutes. Keep broth boiling. Remove chicken breasts when cooked.

Place potatoes in boiling broth and cook until tender. Add corn and chicken back into broth.

Reduce heat to low and stir in the cheese and mix until the cheese is melted.

# Corn and Butternut Squash Chowder

2 tablespoons vegetable oil
1 ½ pounds butternut squash, peeled, seeded and cut into 1-inch cubes (about 5 Cups)
1 medium Onion, chopped
1 package (10 oz) frozen corn kernels, thawed
1 ½ teaspoons curry powder
Salt and pepper to taste
2 Cans (14.5oz each) vegetable broth
½ cup heavy cream

## Directions

In large heavy pot, heat oil over medium-high, add squash and onion. Cook until onion is soft, about 6 minutes. Add corn and curry powder. Cook until curry is fragrant, about 2 minutes. Season with salt and pepper.

Add broth and simmer until squash is tender, about 25 minutes.

In a blender, blend half the soup until smooth.

Return to pot and stir in cream, heat through over medium-low. Do not boil.

## Sweet Potato Soup

2 sweet potatoes
2 white potatoes
1 small turnip
½ cup heavy whipping cream or low fat evaporated milk
6 cups chicken broth
1 tablespoon brown sugar
1 teaspoon ground nutmeg
1 tablespoons butter or margarine
Salt and pepper to taste

### Directions

Peel and cut vegetables into small pieces. Place in a pot, and cover with chicken stock; use only the amount of stock needed to cover. Bring to a boil, and cook until vegetables are tender.

Puree vegetables and liquid in a food processor.

On low heat, return to the pot and slowly stir in the cream, brown sugar, nutmeg, and butter. Add salt and pepper to taste. Do not boil.

# Sweet Pea Soup

2 tablespoons butter
1 medium onion, finely chopped
1 clove garlic, minced
2 cups vegetable stock
3 cups fresh or frozen shelled green peas
salt and pepper to taste
3 tablespoons whipping cream (optional)

## Directions

Melt the butter in a heavy-bottomed saucepan over medium heat. Cook the onion and garlic until tender.

Pour in the vegetable stock and peas, season to taste with salt and pepper. Increase the heat to medium-high, bring to a boil, then reduce heat to low, cover, and simmer until the peas are tender, 12 to 18 minutes.

Puree the peas and liquid in a blender or food processor. Strain back into the saucepan, stir in the cream if using, and reheat. Season with salt and pepper to taste.

## Pumpkin Black Bean Soup

3 (15 ounce) cans black beans,
1 (16 ounce) can diced tomatoes
¼ cup butter
1 ¼ cups chopped onion
3 cloves garlic, minced
1 teaspoon salt
½ teaspoon ground black pepper
4 cups vegetable or beef broth
1 (15 ounce) can pumpkin puree
3 tablespoons sherry vinegar (optional)

### Directions

Drain and rinse 2 cans black beans. Pour the 2 cans of black beans into a food processor or blender, along with the can of tomatoes. Puree until smooth. Set aside.

Melt butter in a large soup pot over medium heat. Add the onion and garlic, and season with salt and pepper. Cook and stir until the onion is softened. Stir in the bean-tomato puree.

Drain and rinse the remaining can of beans. Add rinsed beans, broth, pumpkin puree, and sherry vinegar. Mix until well blended. Simmer for about 25 minutes or until thick enough to coat the back of a metal spoon.

## Crab and Corn Soup

¼ cup butter
¼ cup all-purpose flour
2 cups milk (fat free or whole)
2 cups half-and-half
2 cups whole kernel corn
1 cup chopped onions
1 clove garlic, minced
2 (7 ½ ounce) can crabmeat (drained)
½ teaspoon ground white pepper
½ teaspoon seasoning salt
½ teaspoon of Creole or Old Bay Seasoning™ (optional)
1 tablespoon soy sauce
¼ cup chopped parsley

### Directions

In a heavy-bottomed pot, melt butter, add flour, and stir gently until blended. Do not burn or let it darken. Add milk gradually, stirring continuously. Add half and half, stirring gently while blending. Add corn, onions, and garlic and cook for a few minutes until tender.

Add crabmeat, pepper, salt, and soy sauce and simmer until very hot and small bubbles form around the edge. Do not let it boil. Adjust seasonings to taste. Garnish with sprinkles of chopped fresh parsley when serving and serve hot.

## Vegetable Cheese Soup

1 (15 ounce) can creamed corn
2 cup peeled and cubed potatoes
1½ cup chopped carrots
½ onion, chopped
1 clove garlic, minced
1 teaspoon celery seed
½ teaspoon ground black pepper
2 (14.5 ounce) cans vegetable broth
1 (16 ounce) jar processed cheese sauce

### Directions

In a slow cooker add potatoes, carrots, onion, garlic, celery seeds, and pepper. Add broth and cover, cook on low 8 to 10 hours.

Stir in cheese and corn and cook 30 to 60 minutes or until cheese is melted and blended with vegetables.

# Baked Potato Soup

3 cups peeled and cubed potatoes
½ cup chopped onion
1 can chicken broth
1 teaspoon dried parsley
½ teaspoon salt
1 pinch ground black pepper
2 teaspoons all-purpose flour
1 ½ cups milk
1 ½ cups shredded American cheese
4 slices of bacon, diced

## Directions

In a large stock pot add potatoes, onion, broth, and parsley flakes. Season with salt and pepper. Bring to a boil then and simmer until vegetables become tender.

In a bowl mix flour and milk. Once it is well blended, add to soup mixture and cook on medium to low heat until soup becomes thick.

Stir in cheese and bacon and simmer until cheese is melted.

## Garden Tomato Soup

8 cups chopped fresh tomatoes
1 small onion, diced
2 cloves garlic, minced
6 whole cloves
4 cups chicken broth (vegetarian option: vegetable stock)
4 tablespoons butter
4 tablespoons all-purpose flour
2 teaspoon salt
3 teaspoons white sugar, or to taste

### Directions

In a stockpot, over medium heat, combine the tomatoes, onion, garlic, cloves, and broth.

Bring to a boil, and gently boil for about 20 minutes. Remove from heat. Puree the mixture in a blender or food processor.

In the now empty stockpot, melt the butter over medium heat. Stir in the flour to make a roux. Stir constantly, cooking until the roux is a medium brown.

Gradually whisk in a bit of the tomato mixture, so that no lumps form, then stir in the rest. Add sugar and salt, and fine-tune to taste.

# Chicken and Rice Soup

2 tablespoons olive oil
2 skinless, boneless chicken breasts
salt and pepper to taste
1 tablespoon butter
½ small onion, chopped
2 cloves garlic, finely chopped
3 tablespoons all-purpose flour
10 sprigs Italian flat leaf parsley
3 sprigs fresh thyme
1 bay leaf
3 cups chicken stock
3 cups milk
1 cup water
1 cup uncooked instant rice
1 teaspoon Old Bay Seasoning ™

## Directions

In a large pot, cook chicken in olive oil until juices run clear. Remove chicken, shred and set aside.

Reduce heat to medium-low. Cook onion and garlic in butter until tender. Stir in flour, and cook until lightly browned.

Use twine to tie together the parsley, thyme, and bay leaf. Pour stock and milk into the pot, and stir in the cooked chicken. Place herb bundle into soup. Simmer 25 minutes.

In a separate pot, cook instant rice according to directions. Remove and discard herb bundle from soup. Stir in cooked rice and season with Old Bay before serving.

## Taco Soup

1 packet Hidden Valley Original Mix™
1 packet of Taco Seasoning
1 can Rotel tomatoes
1 can diced tomatoes
1 can each of red beans, pinto beans, kidney beans.
1 pound of ground beef or turkey

### Directions

Brown meat and drain.
In a heavy pot, add all of the ingredients. Do not drain canned ingredients.
Simmer for at least 30 minutes before eating.

# Italian Soup

3 carrots, diced
1 medium onion, chopped
2 cloves garlic, minced
1 teaspoon dried Italian seasoning
4 cups chicken broth
3 tomatoes, diced, or 1 can diced tomatoes
2 cups frozen cheese-filled tortellini
1 (15 ounce) can navy beans, rinsed and drained
grated parmesan cheese (optional)

## Directions

Place the carrots, onion, garlic, Italian seasoning and 2 cups of the broth in a 6-quart saucepot. Heat to a boil.

Reduce the heat to low. Cover and cook for 10 minutes or until the onion is tender.

Add the remaining broth, tomatoes, tortellini and beans. Heat to a boil.

Reduce the heat to low. Cover and cook for 15 minutes or until the tortellini is tender. Serve with grated parmesan cheese, if desired.

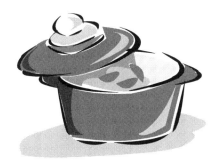

# Comfort Food

The recipes in this section are designed to keep you filled and provide softer foods for you to eat.

It is best to shred meat or cut it into small bite-size pieces to minimize the amount you have to chew.

## Baked Spaghetti

3/4 pound lean ground beef
1 small onion, diced
1 (16 ounce) jar spaghetti sauce
1 pound spaghetti noodles
1 cup shredded mild cheddar cheese
1 cup shredded mozzarella cheese

### Directions

Preheat oven to 350 degrees F (175 degrees C). In large skillet, cook ground beef and onion until brown, drain and return to pan. Mix spaghetti sauce into skillet. Reduce heat and simmer.

Meanwhile, bring a large pot of lightly salted water to a boil. Mix in pasta and cook for 8 to 10 minutes or until al dente. Drain.

Mix together pasta, cheddar cheese and meat mixture, pour into 9x13 pan. Top with mozzarella cheese and bake for 30 minutes, or until heated through and cheese is bubbly.

# Nacho Chicken Casserole

*A great recipe for orthodontic patients to enjoy tortilla chips guilt free.*

1 1/2 cups cooked chicken finely . $,&) &
2 cups crushed nacho-cheese tortilla chips
1 can condensed cream of chicken soup
1/2 cup sour cream
2 tablespoons milk
1 can diced tomatoes with green chilies
1/2 cup shredded part-skim mozzarella cheese
1/2 cup shredded cheddar cheese

## Directions

Preheat oven to 350°.

In a bowl, combine the first six ingredients. Combine the cheeses. Stir half of the cheese into the chicken mixture.

Transfer to a 1-qt. baking dish coated with nonstick cooking spray. Sprinkle with remaining cheeses. Bake, uncovered for 25-30 minutes or until cheese is bubbly.

## Creamy Potato Casserole

6 medium potatoes
1 teaspoon salt
2 cups sour cream
2 cups shredded cheddar cheese
3 tablespoons butter or margarine
3 green onions, thinly sliced
1/4 teaspoon pepper

### Directions

Preheat oven to 350 ° (175 degrees C).

Peel and grate potatoes. Place potatoes in a saucepan with teaspoon of salt and cover with water. Bring to a boil. Reduce heat. Cover and simmer until tender. Drain and cool.

In a bowl, add cooked potatoes, sour cream, cheddar cheese, butter, green onions, salt and pepper.

Transfer to a greased 2-1/2-qt. baking dish. Bake uncovered for 30-35 minutes or until heated through.

Refrigerate any leftovers.

## Ground Beef Casserole

1 ½ lbs. ground beef
1 can tomato soup
1 can mushroom soup
1 onion, chopped
1 8oz. package egg noodles
1 ½ cups grated cheddar cheese
1 can (11 ounces if using a measuring cup) water
Salt & pepper

### Directions

Preheat oven to 350 ° (175 degrees C).

Brown ground beef with onion in large skillet or Dutch oven. Drain and return to pan.

Add mushroom soup, tomato soup and water to ground beef. Add salt and pepper to taste. Simmer for at least 10 minutes.

Cook egg noodles according to directions on package.

In a casserole dish (13 x 9 x 2 or 3 qt.) place a layer of noodles, layer of beef mixture and layer of cheese. Repeat for second layer, noodles, beef and cheese.

Bake 10 to 15 minutes (or until cheese on top is melted).

## Slow Cooker Pot Roast

*You can add carrots, green beans, potatoes or any vegetable of your choice to this recipe to make a complete (and soft) meal.*

2 (10.75 ounce) cans of golden mushroom soup
1 (1 ounce) package dry onion soup mix
¼ cup water
5 ½ pound pot roast

### Directions

In a slow cooker, mix cream of mushroom soup, dry onion soup mix and water. Place pot roast in slow cooker and coat with soup mixture.

Cook on high setting for 3 to 4 hours, or on low setting for 8 to 9 hours.

# Mock Chicken and Dumplings

4 skinless chicken breasts
2 chicken bouillon cubes
1 can cream of chicken soup
1 can cream of celery soup
1 package of flour tortillas 8.5 oz, cut into 2 inch strips

## Directions

In a large Dutch oven, put bouillon cubes and chicken and cover with water. Boil chicken until tender, about 20 minutes. Remove chicken from pot and shred; add shredded chicken back to broth.

Add the soups; bring back to a boil. Drop tortilla strips into boiling soup. Bring back to a boil. Add water if necessary. Reduce heat and simmer until tortillas look like real dumplings.

## Classic Meatloaf

1 ½ pounds ground beef
1 ¼ teaspoons salt
1 egg
1 dash ground black pepper
1 cup soft bread crumbs
½ cup milk
½ cup steak sauce or tomato sauce
1 onion, chopped

### Directions

Preheat oven to 350 ° (175 degrees C). Lightly grease an 8 ½ x 4 ½ inch loaf pan.

In a bowl, combine the ground beef, salt, egg, black pepper and bread crumbs. Pour in the milk, 3 tablespoons of the steak sauce and onion.

Place the mixture into the prepared loaf pan and shape into a loaf. Brush the top with the remaining steak sauce.

Bake 1 hour or until done. Allow to stand 5 minutes before slicing.

## Chicken and Green Bean Casserole

1 tablespoon olive oil
4 skinless, boneless chicken breast, cooked and shredded
1 (14.5 ounce) package of frozen French-style green beans (or 2 canned, drained)
1 (10.5 ounce) can cream of mushroom soup
¼ cup mayonnaise
½ cup sour cream
1 teaspoon garlic powder
¼ cup grated Parmesan cheese

### Directions

Preheat the oven to 350° (175 degrees C).

Heat olive oil in a large skillet over medium-high heat. Cook the chicken breast. Remove from heat, shred and set aside.

Place the green beans into a 2 quart casserole dish. Place the chicken on top of the beans. In a small bowl, mix together the cream of mushroom soup, sour cream and mayonnaise. Spread over the top of the chicken and beans. Sprinkle Parmesan cheese over the top.

Bake for 20-30 minutes in the preheated oven until the cheese is browned.

Serve over noodles, mashed potatoes or rice.

## Ham Potato Broccoli Bake

*This recipe is also good with shredded chicken in place of the ham.*

1 (5.5 ounce) package scalloped potato mix
2 cups boiling water
2 tablespoons butter or margarine
½ cup milk
2 cups cubed fully cooked ham, diced or shredded
1 (10 ounce) package frozen chopped broccoli
1 cup shredded cheddar cheese

### Directions

Preheat oven to 400° (220 degrees C).

In an ungreased 1-1/2-qt. baking dish, combine potatoes with sauce mix, boiling water and butter.

Stir in milk, ham and broccoli. Bake, uncovered 35 minutes or until the potatoes are tender, stirring occasionally.

Sprinkle with cheese. Bake 5 minutes longer or until cheese is melted. Let stand 5 minutes before serving.

# Brown Rice and Black Bean Casserole

½ cup brown rice
1 ½ cup vegetable broth
2 tablespoon olive oil, divided
¼ cup diced onion
1 medium zucchini, thinly sliced
2 skinless boneless chicken breasts
½ teaspoon cumin
salt to taste
ground cayenne pepper to taste
1 (15 oz) can black beans, drained and rinsed
½ cup shredded carrots
1 cups shredded Swiss cheese
1 cup cheddar cheese

## Directions

Preheat oven to 350° (175 degrees C). Lightly grease a large casserole dish. In 1 tablespoon olive oil, cook chicken until juices run clear. Shred and set aside.

Mix rice and vegetable broth in a pot. Bring to a boil. Reduce heat to low, cover, and simmer 45 minutes, or until rice is tender.

In olive oil, cook onion over medium heat until tender. Stir in zucchini, shredded chicken and carrots. Season with cumin, salt, and ground cayenne pepper. Cook until vegetables are tender and chicken is heated through.

In large bowl, mix the cooked rice, onion, zucchini, chicken, beans, carrots, ½ the Swiss cheese and ½ the cheddar cheese. Transfer to the prepared casserole dish, and top with remaining cheese.

Cover casserole loosely with foil, and bake 30 minutes. Uncover, and continue baking 10 minutes, or until bubbly and lightly browned.

## Cornbread Sausage Casserole

1 pound ground pork sausage
1 (16 ounce) package dry corn bread mix
1 (15 ounce) can cream style corn
2/3 cup water
1 medium onion, diced
1 (8 ounce) package shredded cheddar-Monterey Jack cheese blend

### Directions

Preheat oven to 350 ° degrees F (175 degrees C). Lightly grease a 9" x 13" baking dish.

Cook sausage and onion over medium high heat until evenly brown. Drain and set aside.

In a medium bowl, mix corn bread mix, cream style corn and water.

Cover the bottom of the prepared baking dish with about 1/2 inch of the corn bread mixture. Layer with sausage and onion mixture. Cover with cheese. Top with remaining corn bread mixture.

Bake 35 minutes or until a toothpick inserted in the center comes out clean.

Allow to cool 5 minutes before serving.

## Salmon Patties

1 (14.75 ounce) can salmon, drained and flaked
1 small onion, minced
1 egg
½ cup fresh bread crumbs
1 tablespoon Worcestershire sauce
1 ½ teaspoons of Old Bay Seasoning™
¼ teaspoon ground black pepper
¼ cup shredded cheddar cheese
2 tablespoons chopped fresh parsley
1 cup parmesan cheese for coating (can use flour or crackers instead), divided
2 tablespoons canola oil

**Directions**

Preheat oven to 375 degrees. Lightly grease a pan with canola oil.

Combine salmon, onion, egg, bread crumbs, Worcestershire sauce, Old Bay, black pepper, ¾ cup cheese and parsley; mix well. Shape into four patties. Dust lightly with remaining parmesan cheese (or flour or crackers). Chill for 20 minutes.

In the prepared baking pan, bake 20 minutes.

# White Bean Chicken Chili

2 tablespoons vegetable oil
1 pound shredded, cooked chicken meat
1 onion, chopped
2 cloves garlic, minced
1 (14.5 ounce) can chicken broth
1 (24 oz) jar salsa verde
2 (16 ounce) can diced tomatoes
1 (7 ounce) can diced green chilies
½ teaspoon dried oregano
½ teaspoon ground coriander seed
½ teaspoon ground cumin
1 (15 ounce) can white beans
1 (15 ounce) can corn (undrained)
2 tablespoons of corn starch (for thicker chili)
salt to taste
ground black pepper to taste
1 lime, sliced

## Directions

In a soup pot, heat oil and cook onion and garlic until soft.

Stir in broth, salsa verde, tomatoes, chilies, and spices. Bring to a boil, then simmer for 10 minutes.

Add corn, chicken, beans and corn starch; simmer 5 minutes. Season with salt and pepper to taste.

*Topping suggestions*: fresh jalapenos, limes, cilantro, cheese, avocado, or sour cream.

# Chicken Enchiladas with Cottage Cheese

> 1 tablespoon vegetable oil
> 2 skinless, boneless chicken breast cooked and shredded
> ½ cup chopped onion
> 1 (7 ounce) can chopped green chilies
> 1 (1 ounce) package taco seasoning mix
> ½ cup sour cream
> 2 cups cottage cheese
> 1 teaspoon salt
> 1 pinch ground black pepper
> 12 (6 inch) corn or flour tortillas
> 2 cups shredded Monterey Jack cheese
> 1 (10 ounce) can red enchilada sauce

## Directions

**Meat Mixture:** Heat oil in skillet over medium high heat. Brown chicken, shred and set aside. Cook onion with green chilies until tender. Return chicken to pan. Add taco seasoning and prepare meat mixture according to package directions.

**Cheese Mixture:** Mix sour cream and cottage cheese. Season with salt and pepper; stir until well blended.

Preheat oven to 350 ° (175 degrees C).

To Assemble Enchiladas: Heat tortillas until soft. In each tortilla place a spoonful of meat mixture, a spoonful of cheese mixture and a bit of shredded cheese and roll them up.

In a 9"x 13" greased dish, place some of the enchilada sauce. Place rolled tortillas in prepared dish. Top with any remaining meat and cheese mixture, enchilada sauce and remaining shredded cheese.

Bake 30 minutes or until cheese is melted and bubbly.

## Turkey Stroganoff

> 1 pound ground turkey
> ½ teaspoon salt
> ½ teaspoon ground black pepper
> 1 onion diced
> 1 clove garlic, minced
> 4 tablespoons all-purpose flour
> 1 (10.5 ounce) can condensed beef broth
> 1 teaspoon prepared mustard
> 1 (6 ounce) can sliced mushrooms, drained
> cup sour cream
> cup white wine
> salt to taste
> ground black pepper to taste

### Directions

In a large skillet, cook ground turkey, garlic, mushrooms and onion until onion is tender and turkey cooked through. Drain and set aside.

In the empty skillet, mix the flour and beef broth together and bring to a boil, stirring constantly.

Lower the heat and stir in mustard, white wine and meat and onion mixture. Cover and simmer for 15 minutes.

Stir in the sour cream. Heat briefly then salt and pepper to taste.

Serve over egg noodles.

# Tuna Casserole

1 (12 ounce) package egg noodles

2 cups shredded cheddar cheese

1 cup frozen green peas

1 cup frozen corn

2 (6 ounce) cans tuna, drained

2 (10.75 ounce) cans condensed cream of mushroom soup

¼ cup sour cream

¼ cup milk

1 cup crushed potato chips

## Directions

Preheat oven to 400 ° (220 degrees C).

Cook egg noodles as directed on package.

In a large bowl, mix noodles, 1 cup cheese, peas, corn, tuna, soup, milk and sour.

Transfer to a 9x13 inch baking dish, and top with potato chip crumbs and remaining 1 cup cheese.

Bake 15 minutes or until cheese is bubbly.

## Macaroni and Cheese

> 1 (16 ounce) package uncooked elbow macaroni
>
> 1 (16 ounce) container cottage cheese
>
> 1 (16 ounce) container sour cream
>
> 3 eggs
>
> 3 cups shredded sharp Cheddar cheese
>
> ¼ teaspoon salt

### Directions

Preheat oven to 350 ° (175 degrees C). Lightly grease a 3-quart baking dish.

Cook pasta according to package directions, al dente.

In a large bowl combine cooked pasta, cottage cheese, sour cream, eggs, salt and 2 cups cheddar cheese. Mix well and transfer to prepared dish. Top with remaining cheese.

Cover loosely with aluminum foil and bake 30 minutes. Take foil off and bake 10 minutes or until cheese on top is melted.

## Chicken Pot Pie

1 ready-made 9 inch double crust pie
2 cups frozen mixed vegetables
2 boneless, skinless chicken breasts
½ teaspoon dried thyme
1 (10.75 ounce) can condensed cream of
celery soup *or* cream of chicken soup
1 (10.75 ounce) can condensed cream of
potato soup

### Directions

Preheat oven to 400 ° (200 degrees C). Line a 9 inch pie dish with pastry.

Boil chicken to cook. Shred chicken and place in a large bowl.

Blanch frozen mixed vegetables – boil them for 3 to 4 minutes, drain and run cold water over them to stop cooking.

In a bowl, mix together chicken, vegetables, thyme, celery soup and potato soup.

Pour mixture into pastry lined pie dish. Arrange top layer of pie crust, seal and flute the edges. Cut slits in the top of the crust to allow for steam to escape.

Put aluminum foil around the pie crust edges. Bake 30 minutes. Remove foil and continue to bake for an additional 30 minutes until golden brown. Remove from oven and let stand for 5 minutes and then serve.

## Taco Pie

1 tablespoon vegetable oil
1 pound ground turkey
1 cup chopped red bell pepper
1 cup chopped zucchini
1 small yellow onion, chopped
2 cups chopped tomato
1 tablespoon chili powder
1 cup of Spanish rice, cooked to package directions
1 cup Mexican cheese blend
2 (10 inch) burrito-size tortillas

**Directions**

Preheat oven to 350°.

Heat oil in 12-inch skillet over medium-high heat and cook turkey, red pepper, zucchini, onion and chili powder until turkey is thoroughly cooked. Stir in tomato and cook 2 minutes or until tomato is soft. Remove from heat.

Place 1/3 of the turkey mixture in 9-inch deep dish pie plate. Spread 1/3 of the cooked rice on top. Sprinkle with 1/4 cup cheese then top with 1 tortilla. Repeat layers ending with remaining cheese. Bake covered 10 minutes and uncovered for 10 minutes.

Garnish with lettuce, sour cream and chopped cilantro if desired.

# Black Bean Hummus

1 cup canned black beans, drained

1 cup canned garbanzo beans (chickpeas), drained

1 tablespoon olive oil

3 tablespoons fresh lemon juice

2 tablespoons plain nonfat yogurt

2 cloves garlic, roughly chopped

salt and pepper to taste

## Directions

Place black beans, garbanzo beans, olive oil, lemon juice, yogurt, and garlic into the bowl of a blender or food processor.

Season with salt, and pepper. Cover and puree until smooth. Refrigerate until ready to serve.

Serve on toasted pita points or as a sandwich.

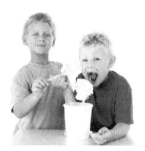

# Desserts

When your teeth are sore it might be a good time to treat yourself to some desserts. They are soft, filling and comforting, so why not?

Included here are some desserts with healthy ingredients and some that are just plain indulgent. Have fun spoiling yourself!

On a gluten-free diet? Baked goods recipes are great made with *Gluten-Free All Purpose Flour.* To use gluten-free flour you also can add xanthan gum to give it that baked-good consistency. All of these ingredients should be at your local grocery store, most of the time in the "Organic" section.

## Pumpkin Muffins

1 (15 ounce) can of pumpkin
3 cups all-purpose flour
2 cups white sugar
2 teaspoons baking soda
½ teaspoon baking powder
2 teaspoons ground cloves
2 teaspoons ground cinnamon
2 teaspoons ground nutmeg
1 teaspoon ground allspice
1 teaspoon salt
1 cup unsweetened applesauce (or vegetable oil)
3 eggs
¼ cup ground flax seed (optional)

**Directions**

Preheat oven to 350° (175 degrees C). Grease 12 muffin cups or line with paper muffin liners.

In a large bowl, stir together flour, sugar, baking soda, baking powder, cloves, cinnamon, nutmeg, allspice, salt and flax seed (if using).

In a separate bowl, beat together pumpkin puree, applesauce and eggs. Stir pumpkin mixture into flour mixture until smooth. Scoop batter into prepared muffin cups.

Bake 20 to 25 minutes, until a toothpick inserted into the center of a muffin comes out clean.

# Banana Muffins

4 ripe bananas, mashed
2 eggs, beaten
¾ cup white sugar
½ cup unsweetened apple sauce
2 cups all-purpose flour
1 teaspoon vanilla
1 teaspoon cinnamon
1 teaspoon salt
1 teaspoon baking soda
1 cup finely ground (in food processor) walnuts

## Directions

Preheat oven to 350 ° (175 degrees C). Grease 12 muffin cups or line with paper muffin liners.

In a medium bowl, combine eggs, bananas, applesauce and vanilla. In a separate bowl, mix together flour, salt, sugar, cinnamon, and baking soda. Stir banana mixture into flour mixture, add walnuts (if desired). Spoon batter into prepared muffin cups.

Bake 20 to 25 minutes, or until a toothpick inserted into center of a muffin comes out clean.

### Strawberry Bread

3 cups fresh strawberries
3 cups all-purpose flour
1½ cups white sugar
2 teaspoons ground cinnamon
1 teaspoon salt
1 teaspoon baking soda
1¼ cups vegetable oil or apple sauce
1 teaspoon vanilla
4 eggs, beaten
1¼ cups ground (in food processor) walnuts or pecans

### Directions

Preheat oven to 350° (175 degrees C). Grease two 9 x 5 inch loaf pans or one Bundt pan.

Dice strawberries, and place in medium-sized bowl. Sprinkle lightly with sugar, and set aside while preparing bread mixture.

Combine flour, sugar, cinnamon, salt and baking soda in large bowl: mix well. Blend oil (or apple sauce), vanilla and eggs into strawberries. Add strawberry mixture to flour mixture, blending until dry ingredients are just moistened. Stir in nuts. Pour into prepared pan(s).

Bake 45 to 50 minutes, or until toothpick inserted comes out clean (may need 15 minutes more in a Bundt pan). Let cool in pans on wire rack for 10 minutes. Turn bread out, and cool completely.

## Easy Pineapple Pudding

> 2 cups fat-free sour cream
> 2 (8 ounce) cans unsweetened crushed pineapple, *not* drained
> 1 (1 ounce) package instant vanilla pudding mix

**Directions**

In a bowl, whisk sour cream, pineapple and pudding mix until blended and thickened.

To create pudding with no chunks, put the mixture in a food processor or blender. Refrigerate one hour before eating.

## Peachy Apple Sauce

10 Red apples, cored and chopped
5 fresh peaches, pitted and chopped
1 teaspoon ground cinnamon
2 tablespoons of brown sugar

### Directions

Put fruit into a slow-cooker; sprinkle with cinnamon. Turn slow-cooker to high. Cover, and cook for 3 hours on high, then switch to low for 2 hours. Stir before serving.

## Custard Bread Pudding

2 eggs
2 cups milk
1 cup sugar
1 tablespoon butter or margarine,
melted
1 teaspoon ground cinnamon
10 slices day-old bread, crusts removed,
cut into ½ inch cubes

**Sauce:**

cup sugar
2 tablespoons all-purpose flour
1 cup water
5 tablespoons butter or margarine
1 teaspoon vanilla extract

### Directions

Preheat oven to 350° (175 degrees C).

In a large bowl, combine eggs, milk, sugar, butter and cinnamon. Add the bread cubes; mix well. Pour into a greased 11" x 7" x 2" baking dish.

Bake 50-60 minutes or until a knife inserted near the center comes out clean.

Sauce: In a saucepan, combine sugar, flour and water until smooth. Add butter. Bring to a boil over medium heat; cook and stir for 2 minutes. Remove from the heat; stir in vanilla. Serve warm or cold over pudding.

## Chocolate Pudding Cake

1 (18.25 ounce) package devil's food cake mix
1 (3.9 ounce) package instant chocolate pudding mix
1 cup sour cream
1 cup milk
½ cup vegetable oil
½ cup water
4 eggs
2 cups mini-semisweet chocolate chips
6 tablespoons butter
1 cup semisweet chocolate chips

### Directions

Preheat oven to 350° (175 degrees C). Grease and flour a 10 inch Bundt pan.

In a large bowl, combine cake mix, pudding mix, sour cream, milk, oil, water and eggs. Beat 4 minutes then mix in chocolate chips.

Pour batter into prepared pan. Bake in the preheated oven 60 to 70 minutes, or until a toothpick inserted into the center of the cake comes out clean.

Cool 10 minutes in the pan, then turn out onto a wire rack and cool completely. Sprinkle the cake with powdered sugar or make the glaze below.

To make the glaze: Melt the butter and 1 cup chocolate chips in a double boiler or microwave oven. Stir until smooth and drizzle over cake.

# Devil Foods Cake with Banana Frosting

1 box Devils Food cake mix
1 (3.5 ounce) package instant banana pudding mix
1 ripe banana, mashed
½ cup milk
2 teaspoons vanilla
1 (8 ounce) container frozen whipped topping, thawed (do *not* use fat free)
¼ cup ice cream hot fudge topping

## Directions

Grease two 9-inch round cake pans. Prepare cake mix according to package. Bake and set aside to cool.

Frosting: In a medium bowl mix pudding, banana and milk until very thick. Gently fold in whipped topping. Spread over any size cake.

Garnish: Put hot fudge topping in a plastic bag. Knead bag and cut a corner off of the bag. Squeeze topping in any pattern you like on top of the cake.

## Vanilla Mousse-Topped Cheesecake

40 vanilla wafers, crushed
2 tablespoons butter or margarine, melted
3 (8 ounce) packages cream cheese, softened, divided
¾ cup sugar
1 tablespoon vanilla and 1 teaspoon vanilla, divided
3 eggs, beaten
1 (8 ounce) tub whipped topping, thawed (do not use fat free or light)
1 (3.5) box of instant vanilla pudding mix
½ cup milk

### Directions

Preheat oven to 350° (175 degrees C).

Mix wafer crumbs and butter; press onto bottom of 9-inch pie pan.

With mixer, mix 3 packages of cream cheese, ¾ cup sugar and 1 tablespoon vanilla until well blended. Slowly add eggs mixing on slow speed. Pour mixture over crust. Bake 50 to 55 min. or until center is almost set. Run knife around rim of pan to loosen cake; cool completely in pan.

Mix pudding, 1 teaspoon vanilla and milk in a large bowl until well blended (will be thick). Fold in whipped topping; spread over cheesecake.

Refrigerate 4 hours before serving, Top with fruit for added flavor.

## Lemon Pound Cake

1 (18.25 ounce) package lemon cake mix
1 (3.5 ounce) package lemon flavored instant pudding mix
1 teaspoon lemon extract
¾ cup apricot nectar*
4 eggs
¼ cup sour cream
½ cup vegetable oil
¼ cup lemon juice
1½ cups confectioners sugar

### Directions

Preheat oven to 350° (175 degrees C). Grease and flour a 10 inch tube pan.

In a large bowl, combine cake mix, pudding, lemon extract, sour cream, apricot nectar, eggs and oil. Mix, then beat on high speed for 3 minutes. Pour batter prepared pan. Bake 60 minutes, or until a toothpick inserted into the cake comes out clean.

To make the glaze: In a small bowl, combine lemon juice and confectioners sugar. Stir until smooth.

Remove cake from oven, and with cake still in pan, pour glaze over top of hot cake, tipping pan to allow excess glaze to run down sides of pan. Allow cake to cool in pan 10 minutes. Remove from pan and cool completely on wire rack.

* *One brand of apricot nectar is Goya. If you have trouble finding it, use apricot juice, Libby's is one brand.*

# CHAPTER 7

## Orthodontic Emergencies

The title of this chapter may be a little misleading because there are so few true orthodontic "emergencies." Included are things that can happen when you wear braces and what you could or should do about these things that happen.

While there is new information here, some of the guidance in this section may seem redundant, but is included in this chapter just in case you see your problem as an emergency.

## A Loose or Broken Bracket

If the bracket is still attached to the braces (the elastic tie should hold it on), then putting a little wax over it should help keep it in place until you can get to the orthodontist's office.

If the bracket comes completely off the tooth, be sure to keep it and bring it with you to your appointment for the repair.

## A Loose or Broken Band

If the band is loose, you can call to see if it is necessary to come in and have it fixed before your regularly scheduled appointment. Do not connect headgear or elastics to any loose bands. You would not want to wait too long for the band to be fixed. If left more than three or four weeks, the space that is created when the band is loose leaves room for bacteria and plaque to enter. If the band is left loose for too long, decalcification can occur, creating permanent white spots the tooth's surface as well as cavities.

It is alright to remove a band until you can go to the orthodontist. If the band is completely off of your tooth it will need to be re-cemented into place.

## A Wire is Broken and Poking

As your teeth align and spaces and gaps close, the wire that connects your braces together, the archwire, can actually grow and feel sharp to your cheeks. You can use clean nail clippers to clip the wire. Or, place wax or a wet cotton ball on the ends of the wire until you can call your orthodontist's office. Usually a quick wire clip the only action required.

## Pain

When you first get braces and after adjustment appointments you may have discomfort. It normally gets better within 72 hours. You can take pain reliever before your adjustments to help head off some discomfort. Other remedies include spraying your mouth with sore throat spray and rinsing with warm salt water.

## Ulcers and Sores in the Mouth

Ulcers and sores can develop while your mouth toughens to its new environment. Once calluses have built up in your mouth, you will hardly notice your braces at all. In the meantime, you can use wax on the area causing the problem. As a note, the less you use the wax the faster your mouth will become used to the braces and the fewer ulcers and sores you will get. This period should not last more than two weeks. If it persists, call your orthodontist to have it looked at.

### A Wire Is Out of the Tube or Slot

If a wire comes out of the tubes, it is fine to attempt to place it back with tweezers. You can also cover the wire with wax and call your orthodontist for an appointment.

### A Metal Tie is Poking

Many orthodontists use elastic ties to connect the archwire to bands and brackets. But if a metal tie is used, it can occasionally be broken from eating or brushing and can start to poke the gums, lips or cheeks. A pencil eraser can be used to direct the wire back to the correct position. If this is not possible or does not work, put a piece of wax over the wire and your orthodontist will repair it at your next appointment.

### Lost Elastic Tie

Call and see what the orthodontist says to do if an elastic tie comes off of your braces. Sometimes it can wait and other times it needs to be replaced more quickly.

## Headgear Does Not Fit Properly

Do not wear headgear that does not fit properly. Call and make an appointment to have the problem fixed.

## Retainer Does Not Fit Properly

If your retainer is too tight, this means you are not wearing it enough. If it is too loose, you should call and have it adjusted as soon as possible. Be sure to seat your retainer firmly and securely in the roof of your mouth, and tell your orthodontist assistant if you are having trouble properly seating your retainer.

## Palatial Expander Appliance is Loose or Has Come Out

You can try pushing the appliance back in place if it is loose. Wax may hold it in place until you can get to an orthodontic appointment. You should call to make an appointment to have it fixed.

If your cemented appliance has come all the way out, do not attempt to put it back. Take care not to lose it and bring it with you to your appointment.

## Swallowing Pieces of Braces or Appliances

The pieces of braces and appliances are not dangerous if swallowed. They should pass through your system normally.

It is *extremely* rare, but if you *inhale* a piece of your braces or appliance, you should see a physician immediately.

## Traumatic Injury to the Face

Take care of the trauma by calling and seeing the appropriate caretaker; 911, the dentist or an oral surgeon. Call your orthodontist as well to discuss the injuries and schedule an appointment.

# Afterword

Looking back on your orthodontic journey in the years to come you will find that it is not the aggravation of the appliances, rubber bands and other braces-related frustrations you most remember. What will stand out in your memory is the moment you looked in the mirror to see the new you.

Having a smile you can be confident and proud of will mean more to you than you could ever realize.

Don't have regrets that you did not do it when you had the chance. Take advantage of this opportunity and work hard, the outcome is *very* worth it.

# Index

*Surviving Braces*

## About the Authors

**Jennifer Webb**
Jennifer has a journalism, advertising and public relations background. She lives in Atlanta, Georgia with her husband and two children.

**Tracy Gilbert**
Tracy has been an orthodontic technician for 32 years. She received her initial training from Dr. Barry Collins in Macon, Georgia. She has since worked for orthodontists in Macon and Atlanta. She has a daughter, Sunny, and resides in Woodstock, Georgia, with her husband, Michael.

---

Ordering Information:

www.jenniferkwebb.com

Email: jennifer@jenniferkwebb.com

Printed in Great Britain
by Amazon

66718433R00095